I PASSED NCLEX! NOW WHAT?!:

A Short Guide to Applying for Jobs

by

T. Writes

Paperback Edition 03/2017
ISBN: 9781542545099

Copyright © T. Writes 2017

T. Writes asserts the moral right to be identified as the author of this work. All rights reserved in all media. No part of this publication may be reproduced, stored in a retrieval system, or transmitted, in any form, or by any means, electronic, mechanical, photocopying, recording or otherwise, without the prior written permission of the author and/or publisher.

I PASSED NCLEX! NOW WHAT?!:

A Short Guide to Applying for Jobs

by

T. Writes

Preface

Hello All! I am excited to share some of my personal experience through the process of stepping into the wonderful world of nursing. This is my first book, so please bear with me. I know my experience may differ from others, but I hope you all find this book to be of some benefit. I wrote this book as a guide I wish I had when I passed NCLEX and began my journey of nursing. A little background about myself is that I have been an RN for slightly over a year. I started off with an Associate's degree in Nursing and have recently earned a Bachelor's degree in nursing. I also have a public health nursing certification. I'm looking to use my experience to help others. I hope this short read will do that plus more. I hope you enjoy!!

Chapter 1: Passing NCLEX

The anxiety that comes after you have taken NCLEX and are waiting that God awful twenty-four to forty-eight hours to login to Pearson and view your results are nerve wrecking. When you enter your login information, pay the quick result fees, and see the lovely green letters of "PASS," it seems the world has rejoiced and the choirs have sung. You cry with joy, especially if it has taken multiple attempts, and think the stress is over. That joy of passing NCLEX will have you on cloud nine and nothing else seems to matter. Take the time to soak in your great accomplishment. YOU HAVE EARNED IT!!! Once you have gloated in your tremendous victory the reality of what's next settles in. The advice that I would give during this stage is to plan, plan, and plan. If I could go back in time, I would have definitely created some sort of outline or plan of the actions to follow after NCLEX. This would have saved me much time and effort. After I passed NCLEX, I just stayed on cloud nine for a lot longer than I should have. The next steps in the process of entering the nursing world as a professional instead of as a student are crucial to success and timing. Congratulations on achieving the first step into entering the nursing world as a nurse!!!

Chapter 2: Job Search Prep

The job search as a new graduate can be overwhelming. There are so many details that weren't discussed throughout nursing school. My advice is to have a mentor or someone that is familiar with the world of nursing. Luckily, I have many family members that are nurses that helped me with figuring things out. As a new graduate, I didn't know what my salary goal should be as I didn't want to seem greedy or feel as if I were being taken advantage of. With the guidance of my family members and doing research, I figured out what my minimum acceptable wage would be, and that helped with setting the standards of my job search.

Another aspect of job searching prep that must be considered is the environment you are seeking to work in. Would you like something fast paced or slow learning environment? I know most new graduates have their eyes set on the big hospital environment. This is a great goal, but is much more competitive. If you are aiming for the hospital environment, you must really stand out as a candidate. This can be done in multiple ways, such as certifications like PALS, ACLS, etc. Some sort of patient care experience also helps you stand out in a hospital candidate pool. New graduate applications for hospitals have hundreds and maybe thousands of applicants. YOU MUST STAND OUT!! Also in the case of getting a hospital job as a new graduate, it is helpful to have connections within the hospital and specifically in the nursing realm. I had many classmates that worked in the hospital as a nursing assistant that were convinced that they would automatically get a job as a nurse when they passed NLCEX and were greatly disappointed when they didn't get the job. The job was given to an outside applicant that was more appealing to the hospital due to having certifications, a bachelor's in nursing, and having some sort of connection within the hospital. It really helps to network as a nursing student when you do clinicals and even with your instructors. They can help you tremendously when it comes to opportunities and connections. As a new graduate nurse with an associate nursing degree, most hospitals I applied to would overlook my application due to the preference of having a new graduate with a bachelor's in nursing. If you have a bachelor's in nursing as a new graduate, it helps you stand out, but still may not guarantee you a job due to the competitiveness of the applicants.

I would recommend setting your goals high, but also thinking about things that you would be willing to settle for or compromise with until you are able to fulfill your high goals. An example of this is me. I applied to every hospital new graduate program I could think of, including a hospital that was close to two hours away from my home. After waiting for a month, I decided I had to look at other opportunities, such as a transitional care facility. I knew that I wasn't fit for a long term care center with regards to working hospice and memory care, but I felt that if I had to choose an area outside of a hospital, I could definitely learn from a transitional care unit. After coming to that realization, I applied to ten or more transitional care centers and units and received six interviews within two weeks of applying. As a new graduate, you must be open and flexible in certain areas in your job search. In due time you will get to the place you really want to be. Don't give up hope. Be willing to gain experience in a different area while waiting for your dream job. While I waited for my dream job of being in the hospital, I worked at a transitional care center which in hindsight was one of the greatest decisions I made. From that work experience, I learned to develop my practical skills and learned the great importance of time management. This greatly prepared me for my current job at the hospital.

Another tip when searching for jobs is to have a baseline for the minimal wages you are willing to accept. From personal experience, they will attempt to pay you at a lower than average wage which is insulting when considering the amount of expenses associated with getting your degree. I started my search with looking at new graduate programs in the hospitals, home care, and transitional care units. There are many transitional care units that are through different organizations that are located in the hospital, which helps with getting a career in the hospital. From my former classmates that took this route to getting a job in the hospital, they spoke of the impact of the references that came from working in the transitional care unit within the hospital. The hospital views these applicants as favorable due to their familiarity with the facility, experience, and familiarity with the complexities of the patients as they have worked with the patients that were previously admitted to the hospital.

Chapter 3: Applying to Jobs and Resumes

As previously discussed, when you have figured out the places you would like to apply to you should really prepare a stellar resume. This is an area that took a lot of time and dedication. My previous careers had nothing to do with nursing, so I had to rethink of creating a resume' to fit nursing. I found great resources on Google and throughout the internet. I followed the formats that were presented online. I eliminated things that had nothing to do with nursing or healthcare and instead emphasized and elaborated on the many skills that I learned throughout nursing school. I also focused on my many experiences throughout my clinicals. I put all of my clinical sites along with the specialty and skills that I demonstrated throughout the clinical experience in the same way you would with a job experience. I also made sure to include at least one instructor as a reference. Be sure to ask for permission before just putting an instructor as a reference. Instructors have been known to decline to provide information as a reference if they weren't asked prior to being placed as a reference on a resume' or job application. Out of respect, please ask instructors and others for permission to list them as a reference. After listing your clinical experiences, emphasize the skills you have learned, such as tube feedings, working with hospice patients, etc. This allows employers to evaluate the amount of training they will have to invest into having you as an employee. If you have experience in the healthcare field, make sure to include that in your resume. I also included my grade point average on my resume', it's not necessary. Rule of thumb is if your grade point average is less than a 3.0 don't include it on your resume. With regards to your objective for your resume, ensure it is something broad. There has been alternating opinions about including your true intentions in the objective. For example, if your end goal is to become a nurse practitioner or an emergency room nurse and you are applying at a long term care facility, they may not hire you due to not wanting to invest in someone that will eventually leave the organization. In my opinion, it is best to leave the objective broad such as "Registered Nurse seeking full time employment and experience in an acute care setting." Tailor your resume to the position you are applying for. I have over ten resumes that were tailored to different positions, especially the new graduate programs. Your resume should speak to your experience, enthusiasm, and willingness to learn and grow as a nurse. This speaks volumes to employers. Before I applied to jobs with my resume, I visited my college's career resource center and had a resume specialist review my resume. This was one of the best things I did! From her critiques, I am able to provide you with the above advice, and it doesn't hurt to have multiple sets of eyes to look over your resume. Speaking of a career resource center, they are a great resource for job search and tips for success. Some schools offer job placement through their career resource center. If you have a career resource center, be sure to check it out!

Chapter 4: Interviews

You have created an awesome resume and have finally got an interview!! First thing to prepare for this interview is to bring copies of your resume, certifications (CPR, BLS, etc.), Nursing License number, and anything else that will be work in your favor. The second thing to prepare for your interview is to bring a list of questions. I brought a notepad full of questions to every interview, and the interviewers were very impressed. Conduct your research of the organization. This will allow you to formulate questions. Some of the questions that I asked during my interviews were:

1. What educational opportunities does your organization offer their staff?
2. Is there any new graduate nursing orientation/ programs to help with developing new nurses?
3. What support are nurses offered through your company?
4. How does your company support nurses pursuing advanced education, such as tuition reimbursement or scholarships?
5. Are there regular continued education opportunities and/ or training? If so, how often?
6. Is there a regularly staffed supervisor on all shifts (this is a question for work environments outside of the hospital)?
7. What is the nurse to patient ratio (this is extremely important to know before accepting a job offer)?

8. How long is orientation and what does it consist of?
9. Ask questions with regards to the organization's mission statement and values.
10. Ask about their organizational connections. For example, if you begin working for a transitional care facility that has partnered with a hospital, you could possibly transfer to the partnered hospital with ease.

It is important to elaborate on your abilities, the expectations of the job, and ask questions to determine if the company would be a good fit for you, especially as a new graduate. As a new graduate nurse, you should feel comfortable and supported with whatever organization you decide to work for. Also, come to the interview prepared to answer questions. I did this be doing a google search of questions asked a nursing interviews. Some of the questions that I was asked were:

How would you resolve a workplace conflict?
How would you deal with an angry family member?
How would you deal with an unprofessional provider?
If you were unclear about a medication, treatment, or care intervention, what would you do?
How would you deal with a nursing assistant or other team member refusing to do something you asked?

Those were the many questions that I was asked. For the most part, the subject of conflict resolution, seeking resources, and dealing with patients and families were the basis of most of the questions. The rest of the steps of preparing for the interview process are pretty much the same as preparing for any other interview. Make sure to dress professionally and arrive early! Another thing to touch base on is there is a possibility that you may have to take a brief test before or after your interview. I was shocked when I had to take short tests for two of my interviews! I passed NCLEX, so I figured that I was done with the testing and demonstrated my nursing knowledge! The tests that I took were very basic. They asked a few questions about frequently used medications, detecting medication errors within doctor's orders, medication calculation, and conflict resolution. The tests were pretty basic and the organization gave me the results of my test shortly after completing the tests. The test also led to the interview questions and allowed for dialogue. I was slightly nervous about the tests, but they were really easy and straight forward. If you passed NCLEX, you will pass these tests and quizzes that some interviews have.

Chapter 5: Preparing and Getting Through Orientation

You rocked the interview and now you've got the job!!! Congratulations!!! This is a big stepping stone into the nursing world. I know you may be filled with some nervousness along with excitement. The next step after getting the job is the orientation process. The orientation process may start off with some classes to get to know the company, their policies and procedures, and nursing skills. The nursing skills are basically a skills day class in which you go over hands on skills and scenarios. During this part of your orientation, come prepared to take notes and don't be afraid to ask questions. This is the perfect time to ask questions and get a feel for the people you may be working with. Make sure you prepare for your orientation by bringing a notebook and pens to take notes.

After the first part of orientation, the next phase is actually shadowing a nurse through the normal work day. Prepare yourself for this stage by showing up in your nursing scrubs, bring your favorite stethoscope, a pen light, scissors, and tons of pens (I also brought a pocket sized nurses reference guide). You will be practicing as a Registered Nurse!!!! This is an exciting and overwhelming time for you, so please be patient with yourself. When I went through this stage at my first nursing job, the on the floor orientation lasted for two weeks. If you have the luxury of having a longer orientation period, be very thankful. If I could go back into time with my orientation, I would have done things differently. When I went into my orientation, I made the mistake of just watching my preceptor do things for a week straight and the last week of my orientation I became more hands on, but still relied heavily on my preceptor. I would not recommend utilizing your orientation the way I did. I was so nervous and afraid that I felt my preceptor would be more qualified to care for patients that I fell into the background. If I could go back into time I would utilize my two weeks in the following ways:

1. The first day of my orientation I would have just sat back and observed everything the preceptor did that day. Ask many questions and carry a small notebook to write notes. Taking notes really helps. I took my small notes and made a quick reference to the daily process which I attached to my name badge. That really comes in handy, trust me!!!

2. The second day of orientation I would have been hands on and led the way. On the second day you should really be taking the lead and having your preceptor at your side as a guide and reference. Also be the one to start charting and writing notes. It will help to have someone by your side to help you structure your charting and notes.

3. The third day of orientation continue with the process of being the leader and having your preceptor as a guide. As things continue to go well, your preceptor will begin to trust you and they will become comfortable with leaving you by yourself. They will be your resource nurse when you have questions.

4. Continue the rest of your orientation as practicing as a nurse and use your preceptor as a resource. I know

the nerves of being new will kick in and scare you. Believe in yourself! Don't be afraid to ask questions. If you aren't sure of something, ask for help. That's what your preceptor is for. Take advantage of them as your resource!

All in all, try your best to be completely hands on throughout the duration of your orientation. You will be well prepared to work independently if you start being hands-on at the beginning of your orientation. Being actively involved and hands on during your orientation also allows your new team to get to know you and you will feel more comfortable coming to your team members for help. During your orientation, you should trial and error different organizational techniques. By doing so, you will be able to figure out what works for you while having a helping hand by your side to help pick up the slack if you fall behind. Orientation is also a great time to learn the process of speaking with providers, whether it be the on-call physician or the attending. Your preceptor will guide you in the structure and process. They will also guide you as to when you should notify the provider. By gaining these experiences during orientation, you will be more equipped to work independently without feeling too overwhelmed. During this experience, expect to make mistakes and be very patient with yourself. You are learning real world nursing which greatly differs from textbook nursing. Be patient and don't beat yourself up throughout the process.

Chapter 6: First Day on Your Own

Orientation is over and now you are on your own as a Registered Nurse!!! The excitement and nervousness can be overwhelming, but remember you can do this! The first day of being on your own and the experiences to follow will shape you as a nurse. Be prepared to show up early and prepared to impact lives. I would recommend, if your institution allows it, that you show up early to gather information about your patients and the tasks you will be doing on your shift. This will help you to be organized and prepared. If any treatments or procedures show up that you aren't familiar with or comfortable with doing, preparing early will allow you to appropriately plan for asking for assistance with that task. By preparing early, you will also allow for time to do research about things that you are unsure of such as medications, tube feedings, etc. Remember that you are new and you will make mistakes. Just try your best to learn from them and not beat yourself up about them. Make some connections and find fellow nurses that you feel comfortable with as far as asking questions. Remember nursing is a team-oriented field and we must be team oriented. When things become overwhelming, don't be afraid to ask for help and voice your concerns.

Author's Note

Thanks for reading this short guide. This is my first book and I would greatly appreciate feedback. I created this due to when I graduated there weren't many resources or books that touched on the topic of the actions to take after passing NCLEX. Feel free to email me any comments, concerns, suggestions, and questions to Twritesliterature@gmail.com. Again thanks so much for your attention and I hope this guide helps you get your first awesome nursing job.

www.ingramcontent.com/pod-product-compliance
Lightning Source LLC
Chambersburg PA
CBHW070721210526
45170CB00021B/1401